I0440076

Honey, Are You For Real?

Exposing and Challenging Claims and Labels of "Real Honey" and "The Best Honey"

By Ruth Tan

All Copyright 2013.

All rights reserved. No part of this publication may be reproduced, stored in a retrieval system, or transmitted in any form or by any means, electronics, mechanical, photocopying, recording or otherwise, without the prior permission of the publication.

Prologue

Was there ever a point in time that you felt besieged by the barrage of terms such as "natural honey", "pure honey", "creamy honey", "real honey", "raw honey" which left you with too many questions to form an informed opinion on which honey to buy, or have you ever wondered what was this "real honey" or "the best honey" that so many people were talking about? If yes, this book is for you.

This book is passionately written for those who seriously want to find out more about how to choose honey, and how to make sense of the various commercial labels, names, claims related to honey and for those who wish to clear the misconceptions and myths revolving honey. It is for all who genuinely feel that the sweetener means something to them and are eager to discover more facts that can help them make smarter buying decisions.

I have crossed the paths of those who want to buy honey after learning from others that eating honey is good but are not prepared in the slightest to get more information on the bottles of honey they buy. Past observations also revealed that many customers would happily buy bottles of Manuka honey labeled with only a Total Activity number (ie no UMF certification at all) from honey stores whose walls are splashed with articles on the importance of choosing Manuka honey with the UMF label . (It is atrocious how honey sellers are preying and thriving on the ignorance of consumers.) Some people told me that they were too lazy to read long stories and instructions about honey. There was once I asked a young, educated lady about the honey that she had been consuming daily at home for months. She was unable to tell the brand of the honey. Some people told me that they just wanted to get the cheapest bottle and anything else wouldn't matter, not even the taste. (I appreciate their honesty.) "Well, all honey is sweet right, isn't it?" So they dismissed it very quickly and immediately alienated themselves from any further clarification by anyone. (I don't appreciate the low value placed on honey by these people.)

So, if your interest level is limited only to "honey is just honey, so just give me any honey", the information offered in this book would not mean much to you. But if you are surprised that not all honey is equal, and are intrigued to find out more, this book will not disappoint you. The exposing of lying labels, bogus claims and deceptive and misleading marketing promises will give you a completely new pair of eyes to see and weigh the honey bottles you find on the shelves.

This book contains truths that came to me bit by bit as revelations over several years as I encountered more and more types of honey and learned from honey lovers and beekeepers from all over the world especially via the hugely popular benefits-of-honey.com platform. "I should have known this earlier!" was a reaction each time I experienced something new about buying honey. More people should know that there is no commercial standard or definition of real honey and that they cannot rely just on marketing claims and labels to understand the honey bought.

Now let's cast some light on this golden liquid. Hold tight and be prepared for some glaring truths.

Table of Contents

So Many Types of Honey! Which to Buy?

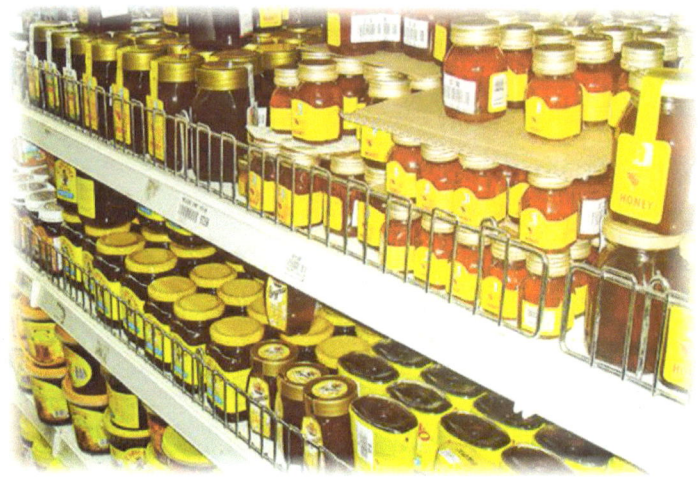

"Which honey to buy?", "Which honey is best?", "Which brand shall I buy?", "What's the difference between pure honey and raw honey?", "Is raw honey or organic honey more superior?', "Is local honey better?" - These are probably the most frequently asked questions from people who have just discovered honey and want to know which bottle of honey to pick. I wish life were simple enough for me to address all these queries in a sentence or two. I'm afraid it isn't. Nevertheless, let's get the most common terms "raw", "local", "pure", "organic" clarified here.

Local Honey versus Foreign Honey

Where can I buy good quality honey? Experience tells that honey is aplenty everywhere, but good quality honey can be rare in some countries. Ideally, get fresh local honey directly from credible sources, bee farms and trusted beekeepers. Don't get me wrong, I have nothing against buying honey from overseas (I do that a lot), but what I am saying is – remember to support your local beekeepers!

Local honey comes from the bees that live in your neighborhood and is well known to be a great immune booster against seasonal allergies. Also by buying local honey, it is easier to ensure what you eat is 100% pure, unadulterated, and find out if it's raw and organic, without even understanding fully what those terms mean. And if you have the zest of going the extra mile to trace the source of the food you eat, pose questions about the honey quality, request a farm visit from your beekeeper and witness for yourself the whole process of harvesting the honey, including extracting, filtering and bottling.

Imported, foreign honey can be much cheaper than local honey, and this makes it extremely hard for small local beekeepers to compete with the big honey suppliers who are exporting in huge volumes to different countries. But beware, some foreign honey is now locally packed and sold as "local honey". For instance, America imports a lot of honey from China to repackage and some suppliers label it as their local products. Nonetheless, I reckon it's not an easy subject to deliberate when the harsh reality of life sets in and cuts deep. While the small beekeepers find it ridiculous to sustain pleasures in beekeeping when confronted with dire livelihood issues, consumers feel it's impossible to support relatively more expensive local honey with their limited spending power.

Did you Say Commercial Honey Is Worth Buying!

Raw honey is unprocessed, unheated, and thus highly valued for its live enzymes which are significantly destroyed in preparing pasteurized honey. However, if bee farms and beekeepers aren't within any possible reach for you and accessing the freshest raw or any local farmers' market is out of the question, then regular, commercial honey from the stores and online shops would probably be what you are looking at. Now those who have been screaming "DO NOT buy grocery store-brand honey" would probably be appalled by the statement I just made.

Living in an urban food desert, where the agricultural sector is virtually absent and almost all fresh produce, including honey, is imported, I hold on to the belief that we eat the best that is known and available to you, at a price that we can afford. How many people can actually afford to eat "honey fit for the kings and ministers"? It's incredible that even a commodity like honey (or is it not anymore) has to end up in a place of scrambling for the most premium spots in the market. It's mind-blowing to realize that consumers can actually end up paying an indecent amount for intense marketing and research just to have prestigious institutions and labs prove and certify that certain honey is of a more superior quality or offers more health benefits than the regular.

An online news portal reported that an old man from the UK cured his chronic eye infection of eight years with a 99p jar of supermarket honey. He had spent a fortune on visiting doctors and eye specialists and had a whole fridge full of eye drops but none had worked. Then he stumbled across the honey cure while on a trip to Jerusalem, Israel and applied the honey on his eyelid and tear duct twice a day. In just a few weeks, the painful infection cleared up completely. I'm neither trying to promote supermarket honey nor suggest that supermarket is just as good as honey directly bought from the farms. What I am getting across is, supermarket honey may not be the best choice, but there is something very precious in honey which the bees have deposited that tells is not to dismiss supermarket honey so quickly.

The idea of eating honey is about replacing as much refined sugars as possible in your diet. Where beekeepers are not within reach, 100% pure honey from the store is still better off than refined sugar. The same logic applies when comparing other sweeteners - one would be far better off with table sugar than high fructose corn syrup or any artificial sweetener. So, isn't it better for people who have zero access to beekeepers and bee farms to eat certain honey or not to eat at all, taking into account the fierce onslaught of today's highly refined sugar, high fructose corn syrup, and artificial sugars? And considering the nature of man or should I just say how all economies in the world are run, we will never see the day when everyone in this world, rich and poor, get to eat the most luxurious quality honey in this world at the price of commodities. There was a European beekeeper who tried to hard sell me the "purest honey" from his farm. I probably cheesed him off by suggesting that he could look into how he could help take care of the locals first, keep his purest honey and help make honey accessible and affordable to the locals. As I meet more and more beekeepers from all over, the concern about maximizing profit (not just survival issues) is extremely real. I'm not trying to be judgmental here, but different people do see honey with very different eyes. There are many beekeepers whose love for bees exudes through and through and supersedes any interest in the health benefits of honey, and also those who are single-mindedly focused on the pure desire to prosper a business by keeping bees. And, rarely, I also meet beekeepers who stop talking to me about beekeeping after realizing that I know nuts about it, but continue to freely and passionately share with me about the benefits of honey.

Not All Honey Is Equal

Isn't honey just honey? No, with the diverse beliefs and practices in beekeeping all over the world, all honey is not created equal, and not when it has gone through the multiple layers and channels of the distribution system. We have to understand that not all honey is "created" equal. Multiple factors related to the floral source of the honey can affect the quality of honey, for instance floral varietals, weather, soil, landscape, environment pollution level (e.g. New Zealand boasts exceptionally low levels of environmental pollution for beekeeping operations). Also, making choices on which honey to buy can be complicated for consumers when so many beekeepers from different parts of the world are shouting unverifiable claims that their honey is the best and the purest in the world. Beekeeping practices, ethics, culture, and legal policies in the country (eg the administration of sugar syrup and antibiotics to bees, the type of bee smoker used for calming the bees), etc. are all determinants of honey quality. In certain countries, it is a norm and a widespread practice for beekeepers to feed their bees with sugar.

While all honey floral varietals are good, not all are equal in terms of medicinal value. Some honey varieties have more medicinal value and are coveted much more than others due to its higher anti-bacterial properties, for instance, New Zealand's well-acclaimed medihoney or Manuka honey, among which is the most coveted hospital grade UMF 20+ for treating infected and gangrenous wounds, Australia's Jarrah honey,

Malaysia's Tualang honey, Yemeni Sidr honey and European honeydew honey. Such varietals of honey are tagged 10 or 20 times more in price than regular honey and are simply beyond the reach of many consumers' purchasing power. So, these expensive varietals are usually not consumed on a daily basis but kept as a treasure for treating burns, cuts, coughs, sore-throats, infections, and other ills. But of course there are people who somehow believe only in Manuka and consume it daily (and have tried to convince me that that is the only honey worth eating). Some other honey varietals also have their own unique factor, e.g Buckwheat honey is high in iron content, Eucalyptus honey has good calming effects, etc.

There's the relatively scarce and more expensive organic honey for those who believe in eating only the purest form of this natural sweetener - 100% free of pesticides or environmental pollutants, whereby the nectar and pollen sources consist essentially of organic crops as the origin of bees and locations of apiaries are regulated by a strict set of guidelines. Whether it has to be organic honey depends on whether you are an ardent believer of organic foods as a whole. For honey to be certified organic, the manufacturer has to meet a set of stringent organic standards and conditions during the honey production (set by a organic agriculture certification body), which include source of the nectar, honey bees foraging area, bees management, honey extracting process, transportation, processing temperature, and packaging materials. Go for organic honey if you feel that it's worth paying extra for a healthier choice and you can have the peace of mind by eating honey that has been tested and guaranteed to be free of any residues of pesticides or environmental pollutants.

Endless Honey Floral Varietals, Each with a Distinct Taste of its Own

Purity assumed, "palate" or personal preference for taste is perhaps one of the most important considerations in deciding which honey is "the best". If you are not satisfied with eating floral-blend honey of unidentified floral varietals, then explore the mono-floral varietals. Choose a floral varietal that goes down well with you especially if you are taking direct or mixing it with just water for daily consumption. Taste can be very subjective and personal, so not every variety is going to wow everyone. Like enjoying and appreciating wine, everyone has their unique take when it comes to tasting this golden liquid. Some prefer it heavy-bodied and robust while others, blend and mild. For instance, New Zealand's Active Manuka Honey has a huge fan base, but it's not always a big hit with everyone. For some people, it tastes like medicine (it's actually known as Medihoney in some pharmacies!). It takes an acquired taste for some to love it.

If you are using honey in your beverage and other foods, experiment with get a few varietals, do some trial and error to see how combinations of food and honey types work for you. Generally, for food or dishes with very distinct, strong taste, go for a mild light taste honey, whereas for food that is blander, you can try a stronger honey to create a tastier concoction, e.g English breakfast tea tastes a world of difference when a flavorsome honey such as a Leatherwood , Buckwheat, or Eucalyptus floral varietal is added to it. But of course, if you are prepared for a more adventurous experience with honey, you can break all rules and combine any type of honey with any type food. Possibilities with honey flavor nuances are never-ending. There exist thousands of different floral plant genera with thousands of distinct species and hybrids. Different countries yield their own delicious floral varieties of honey in various sets of farming conditions - environment, weather, soil, and honeybee species, with many claiming to produce the best honey, the finest, and most exquisite honey in the world. Whatever the flavor, and whatever the aroma, so long as the honey produced is 100% pure, unadulterated, untainted by any chemicals or pesticides, it is as good as gold.

Veiled in this fragile filigree of wax is the essence of sunshine, golden and limpid, tasting of grassy meadows, mountain wildflowers, lavishly blooming orange trees, or scrubby desert weeds. Honey, even more than wine, is a reflection of place. If the process of grape to glass is alchemy, then the trail from blossom to bottle is one of reflection. The nectar collected by the bee is the spirit and sap of the plant, its sweetest juice. Honey is the flower transmuted, its scent and beauty transformed into aroma and taste.
~ Stephanie Rosenbaum

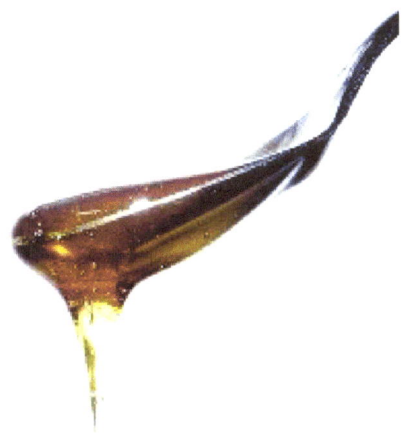

Honey comes in creamed/semi solid and liquid forms. While creamed honey is mess-free and favored by those who enjoy using honey as a spread for toast, liquid honey is an all-time favorite for drizzling over pastries, pancakes, biscuits, and fresh greens. Hence, which honey is considered to be "the best" is also partly dependent on how one prefers to apply or eat honey.

In addition, honey is color graded into light, amber, and dark categories which do not really have any bearing on quality. Some of the most distinctively and strongly flavored honey varieties, such as basswood, are very light, while very mild and pleasant honeys such as tulip poplar can be quite dark. Honey color is measured on the Pfund Scale in millimeters. While it is not an indicator of honey quality and there are exceptions to the rule, generally speaking, the darker color the honey, the higher its mineral contents, the pH readings, and the aroma/flavor levels. Minerals such as potassium, chlorine, sulfur, iron, manganese, magnesium, and sodium also have been found to be much higher in darker honeys.

Eat the Best of What's Within Your Reach and Means

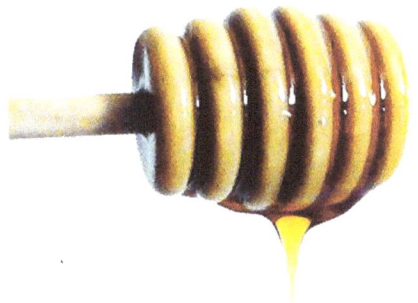

A final note on which honey to buy - I believe in eating the best of what you can find and afford. There are people who don't react in the friendliest way when they discover I'm a honey enthusiast: "Sorry, I don't eat honey because I can't afford it." What can I say? I believe you would agree with me that it is a totally valid reasoning. (That is why so many countries which are not as affluent use honey only as a medicine and consuming it for pleasure or using it as a health supplement for better body immunity are just not part of their culture.) There have also been honey suppliers who tried to sell me certified honey that is "fit for the kings and minsters" and of course at an exorbitant price (which I shall not disclose here because it's going to sound like extortions for most people.) Well, I can't comment too much on this because I am not of that royal league. But what is price when the worth of honey cannot be appreciated? Should I care what some beekeepers are charging for their honey? Honey is too precious to be wasted on anyone, rich or poor, who can't see its value.

I love exploring the different floral varietals of honey. At any one time, I can have more than ten opened bottles of honey in my kitchen. Chinese honey can be very interesting in terms of its aroma and taste, but I must say after so many fraud cases related to foods from China, I am pretty wary of it. If you are buying from overseas, look for floral varietals that are abundant in the country. For example, if you are in Taiwan, consider getting longan and lychee honey because of there is a great flow of longan and lychee flower nectar in the country. And you might want to check on the authenticity when picking up a bottle of peach honey because there is a very limited amount of nectar from the peach flowers in Taiwan. The possibility of getting an adulterated or artificially peach-flavored honey is higher than in the USA or Japan. Beware, there are too many bottles of honey on the shelves that contain food additives and flavor enhancers, so make sure your blackberry honey, blueberry honey, orange honey and lychee honey really originate from the nectar of the respective blossoms and are not added with any flavoring or fruit essence.

So, your choice of honey really depends on a combination of factors such as price, affordability, accessibility to beekeepers and trusted commercial brands, how much you believe in the health and healing benefits of honey, and how far you are willing to go in pursuing good sugar and getting to the bottom of the source and quality of the honey. At the end of the day, my opinion is, even if raw honey is unavailable, commercial honey can still be many times more superior to refined table sugar, high fructose corn syrup and any artificial sugar. I'm not against buying cheap honey, but I would say think twice and double check, because it's all too easy to find fake or adulterated honey sold at the price of rare floral varietals such as Corsican honey, but just impossible to get quality pure honey at the same low price as corn syrup.

UMF Manuka's Big Price Tag

So what is so special about UMF Manuka honey?

We all know all types of honey produce an antiseptic molecule called hydrogen peroxide which is derived from glucose oxidase, an enzyme added by the bees. However, one floral varietal called Manuka differentiates itself with an additional antibacterial prowess for treating cuts, burns, stomach ulcers, skin infections and more. I'm certain that there are also other indigenous varietals that have an exceptionally high medical value in various parts of the world, but New Zealand's Manuka is probably the best known medicinal varietal because of the unmatched amount of attention given in terms of empirical studies and research, accreditation and certification since 1982.

For decades, - the prestigious, expensive registered trademark Unique Manuka Factor (UMF) dominated the market even though many suppliers tried to trick consumers with similar labels such as UMP, UMV, etc. It was well known that some non-peroxide activity (NPA) was present in Manuka honey, but nobody knew what the system of UMF actually quantified and measured until the MGO labeled Manuka honey finally made its appearance in the market in 2008 and revealed to the world that Methylglyoxal was the mysterious ingredient responsible for the exceptional anti-bacteria action of Manuka honey. Supposedly, the higher the MGO level in honey, the greater the antimicrobial effect and MGO 100+ is the equivalent of UMF 10+. However, UMF Manuka products are still able to command a much higher price than Manuka indicated with MGO or NPA levels. For instance, a bottle of UMF 20+ can cost more than twice the price of a bottle with NPA 20+. And because the average Joe and Jane only recognize the label "Manuka", the huge price differential in Manuka products has led to much confusion and misunderstanding.

The UMF association has claimed that due to the complex interactions with other components in honey, MGO, unlike UMF, does not directly correspond with the degree of antibacterial strength. Thus MGO 400+ is actually not the equivalent of UMF 40+, but UMF 20+. Much as UMF proponents have tried to influence me and get me to endorse just the UMF label by insisting that the UMF label is the best measure of Manuka's healing ability, my stance remains that the choice of honey for anyone is all about weighing factors related to assurance, individual's importance placed on certification, and price. When you know that there are people who would love to eat honey but cannot afford to do so, you can't help but to have a different perspective of branded foods, including extensively certified, exorbitantly priced honey which is not within the reach of everyone.

Please don't get me wrong, go ahead and look for the UMF Manuka label by all means. I am not trying to put down commercial trademarks or write off laboratory testing and certification of honey because they can mean assurance which gives consumers peace of mind, but when the honey ends up being so costly and luxuriously exclusive, and becomes far beyond the means of the masses to benefit from, no matter how superb the food is as a medicine, it bears little relevance to the average consumer.

Two Most Favorite Words of Honey Suppliers – "Pure" and "Natural"

Commercial honey is labeled as natural honey, pure honey, raw honey, pure natural honey... the list continues. It takes me by no surprise that honey, like any other products, is not spared from ambiguous labeling by suppliers. There is absolutely no standard on what constitutes honey. With so many different claims of honey on the shelf, we often land up confused and unsecure about how much authentic honey and counterfeit honey we are consuming. Here, I would like to list and share a few questions that many people have raised to illustrate the issue.

"I see so many different claims and labels of honey in the shop. What does the term "pure honey" actually mean?"

"Pure honey" can be taken to mean "100% unadulterated honey with no other contents (for instance, water, sucrose) added", or at least this would be what I think honey suppliers would hope how consumers read. However, to be on the critical side, I would not rule out the possibility that "pure honey" simply means "real honey" and thus the product may contain "real honey" in an unknown amount not necessarily equivalent to 100%. Whatever it is, the term "pure honey" can be ambiguous and even misleading.

Can I assume that "natural honey" means "unpasteurized honey"?

I don't think so. While honey retailers may wish that consumers would associate or even equate the "natural honey" label with meanings of "unpasteurized honey" or "raw honey", the fact is the "natural" label on honey does not render it any more special than other honey. A lot of commercial honey, even when it's labeled as "natural", is treated with heat and filtered (microscopic particles and pollen in honey removed) to slow down crystallization and keep the jars presentable on the shelves. (Ironically, speckle-free honey is somewhat perceived as good quality honey and even "pure" by most consumers.)

Raw, unfiltered honey is now mostly directly purchased from the local honey farms, which do not exist in places within easy reach for some consumers. Every country has its own regulations regarding the "pasteurized" labeling; for some countries, the term "unpasteurized" label on honey is prohibited, but you can sometimes find the label "raw" instead.

Since cream honey appears more concentrated, is it then better than liquid honey?

Form is not a factor in judging the nutritional value of honey. Cream honey, which is formed by allowing the honey to granulate at a controlled temperature of about 55 degree Fahrenheit, can be better in terms of convenience for some consumers who find it less messy to spread the honey over toast, biscuit, whereas liquid is better for drizzling over pancakes, waffles, etc. and mixes easily with water or foods such as vegetable salads.

Finally, my favorite personal quote which sums up my sentiments regarding purity of honey:

"I believe the best labs can create synthetic liquids that look and taste like real honey and even have the same glucose-fructose molecular structure, but NEVER can they fake something that works the same as real honey for our health and well-being. Because the bees have added a MYSTERIOUS GOODNESS of their own that can never be comprehended by the most ingenious mind or counterfeited by the most advanced technology." ~ Ruth Tan

"Pure" and "Raw" – The Big Mix-up

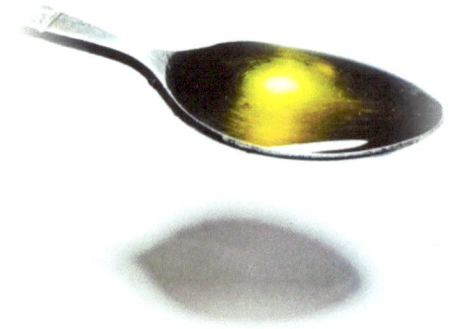

Honey is to best eaten raw and unprocessed. Hence whether the honey one has purchased is raw or heated becomes a concern of consumers. However, the irresponsible use of the term "pure" by honey marketers and sellers have added to the confusion about the concepts of "pure honey" and "raw honey" and the difference between the two.

I've seen many honey sellers making this claim – "pure honey contains pollen and active enzymes". "Pure honey" here seems to mean "raw, unfiltered honey"! While honey with pollen is not filtered in the bottling process, it does not mean it is also definitely pure, 100%, unadulterated. Similarly, it does not mean that unheated or lightly heated honey with active enzymes is surely pure. The term "pure" is so loosely used that the intentions of honey suppliers in describing their honey are no longer easy to read and understand. Remember, "pure honey" may not necessarily be raw honey and "raw honey" may not necessarily be pure honey. Even raw honey with pollen can be contaminated with antibiotics or lead. There seems to be more heated debates and controversies about whether filtered, pollen-free honey should be called real honey than whether enough checks and tests have been done to protect consumers from imported honey that has been treated and contaminated with harmful chemicals. This, I find it really strange.

Heating and Filtering Myths

We are all concern about whether honey we buy has been heated or raw as heat can lead to enzymatic destruction. Heat is relative. For those living in tropical countries, 30 degree Celsius can be "cool", while the same temperature may be "hot" for those from a temperate climate. Any alteration of honey in terms of quality and floral aromatic deterioration is an outcome of temperature and time, for instance, storing honey at a temperature of 35 degree Celsius for three months can result in the same degree of damage as storing it at 40 degree Celsius for one month. In colder climates, it is common for beekeepers to apply heat to extract honey easily from their hives and out of the frames. When honey is said to be "cold extracted", no heating is involved in the honey extraction. Similarly, because honey candies quickly during the bottling, heat is applied to make the honey less viscous for easy bottling.

Customer-focused honey sellers would ensure the bare minimum amount of heat necessary for bottling. For instance, some honey sellers would never treat their honey with a temperature higher than 45 degree Celsius, which is lower than what the hive generates in the hot summer season. Beekeepers harvesting honey in warm climates usually do not encounter the same heating and bottling issues. The viscosity of most honey varietals is not as high and heating is usually not required. Thus, for most commercial honey in Asia, "raw" labels are hardly ever seen on honey bottles because there is simply no necessity to heat the honey to resolve crystallization, extracting and bottling issues.

It's a common belief that most honey you find in the retail stores is typically treated at 70 degrees Celsius to make it flow rapidly and facilitate the filtration and bottling process. "Pasteurization" is often the term used by these retailers to refer to this heating and suggested as a beneficial process for consumers, just like how it is claimed in milk and other dairy products that pasteurization purifies and kills spoilage organisms. But honey is a supersaturated liquid that does not support the breeding of bacteria. And those who cite the risk of infants getting botulism from honey as a rationale for pasteurization also do not have a case because pasteurization will not destroy botulism spores. Children less than 18 months old are susceptible to infant botulism and should not be fed raw agricultural products of any kind. The point is, don't give honey to babies. As for the rest of the people, give us unpasteurized, raw honey in all its full goodness.

Commercial Lie or Consumer Irony

The Big Controversy: Who Wants Filtered Honey?

Have you ever heard how some consumers and honey suppliers have argued over filtered honey?

Voice of Consumers:

Don't fool us, just give us real honey of the best quality, I don't want anything processed. I want only the best. Retain all the goodness in honey, don't process it, don't treat it, give me the most original, raw, pure and unadulterated honey.

Voice of Honey Suppliers:

Whether filtered or unfiltered honey, it is all consumers' wish. We can do both. When I offer unfiltered raw honey, nobody buys. Crystallization makes honey look like processed sugary grains. Filtering and pasteurization slows down the crystallization process and makes the honey stable and looks clear and delicious on the shelves. I know you like the most original honey with the nutritious pollen inside, but if I don't filter my honey, you cannot accept it. You see the wax particles and pollen as dirt and label my honey as impure. I reckon that you like only clean and clear honey. The aesthetic value of honey matters much to you. I'm just giving you what you want.

Your Verdict as a Consumer?

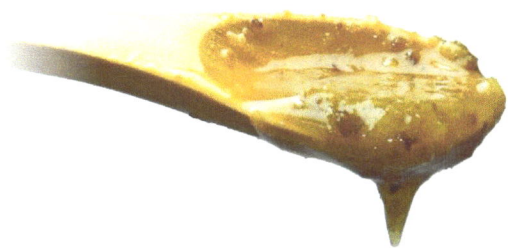

For most consumers, good quality honey is expected to be visually free of debris - clean and clear. Honey which is high in pollen content appears cloudy. The presence of many other "ingredients" such as particles of wax, bees, splinters of wood, and dust also makes it look unappetizing and unappealing for consumers to buy and consume. Unfortunately, no matter how wholesome or how much health benefits some of these particles like pollen can offer, many consumers are more ready to associate them with contaminants and impurities than raw and unprocessed honey and thus immediately reject them at the store. (If you are one of those who would love to see bee legs and wings in their tea added with honey, I believe you are far from being the majority.) And this explains why it's almost impossible to find unfiltered, raw honey on the shelf. Its cloudy appearance makes them commercially unviable. What a sorry irony.

To make things even more complicated for consumers, some honey suppliers market their honey by claiming that their honey is only "strained" and never "filtered". With no explanation on the terms, the average consumer will never know the difference. Many will not even ask more and simply trust that the honey quality is good as long as the honey supplier appears to know what he or she is talking about. Amongst beekeepers who differentiate the two terms, most seem to agree that straining involves only removal of whole bees, bees parts, wax chunk and big particles, whereas filtering removes fine particles including pollen. And there are those who classify their honey as only minimally filtered, so apparently there are different sizes of filters with varying levels of ability to remove substances in the honey.

It's a never-ending debate unless consumers become more educated about unfiltered and crystallized honey and accept dirty-looking honey. Who is going to invest in educating the consumers? Now there seems to be nobody. Perhaps some honey regulatory body or non-profit association in future. But all this is going to take time. I hope this book will serve its purpose in correcting the misconceptions of honey consumers, which in turn would thwart marketers' efforts in using misleading and false honey claims and labels and eventually trigger a push for the authorities to look into the setting of basic standards on honey quality, claims and labels.

World of Honeycombs

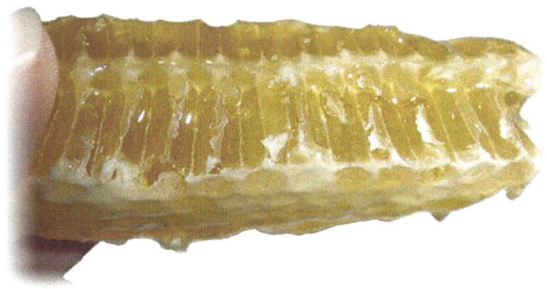

Honeycombs are a favorite theme of many foods, including chocolates, candy, cakes, and even sugar. Perhaps manufacturers know consumers can't help but to immediately associate the symmetrical cells of refined sugar with positive, wholesome notions of sweetness, health, and nature.

Here are several foods made to look just like honeycombs and of course, you probably have more to suggest. Totally awesome and incredibly mouth-watering looking stuff, but some of these have a tremendous amount of empty calories present in them and are rejected as junk by the health-conscious. And remember, they do not bear any of the health benefits that honeycomb promises.

1. Candy Bar

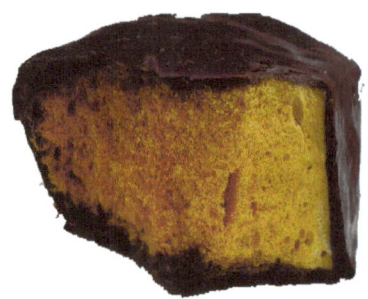

An absolutely crunchy and crumbly candy mimicking the honeycomb pattern and coated with milk chocolate. A hit amongst teens!

2. Malay Cake, Ambon

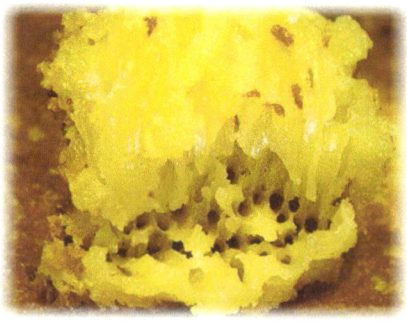

A rich Malay traditional cake made of coconut milk, sugar, and egg. The gorgeous, elastic texture is a big draw.

3. Chocolate

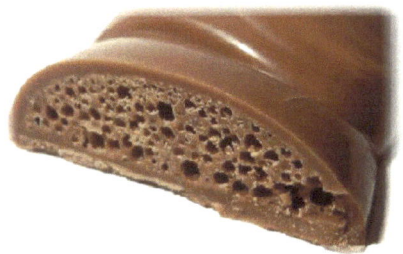

The honeycomb-like aerated portions of this chocolate is soft, fragile, melts in the mouth. A highly addictive snack amongst the sweet-tooth!

4. Rock Sugar

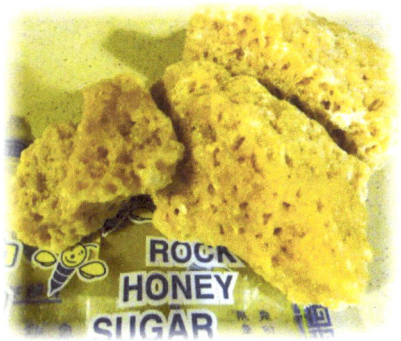

Refined and processed cane sugar which is popularly used as an ingredient in many Chinese traditional sweet desserts, soups and cakes. It may be labeled as "rock honey sugar" but there is absolutely no honey in it.

5. Honeycomb Cereal

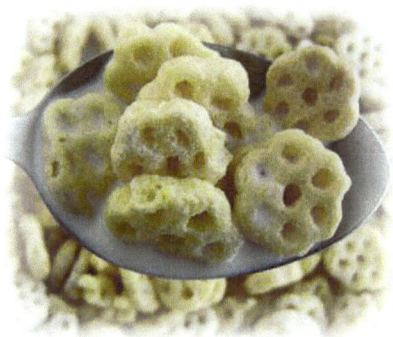

A honey-sweet taste corn and oat cereal that contains no honey but has become an addictive breakfast choice of many children and adults alike.

Innovative Bee Products - Pure Honey Drops

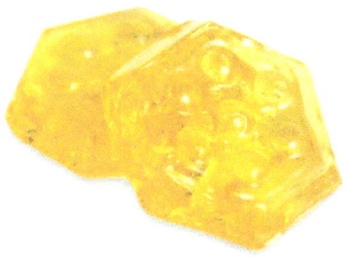

I am amazed by how the innovativeness of honey suppliers has influenced the presentation of honey related products these days. First came honey packed and sealed in tiny plastic containers (5ml), then honey sticks for kids, honey powder for baking, and even honey bottled in exclusive fanciful bottles. And to compete directly with the all too familiar sugar cubes, there are now honey cubes that are marketed as "honey that you can hold", "the world's first 100% pure, non-messy honey cube for tea and coffee drinkers."

Out of plain curiosity, I got hold of some of these honey drops to try and would like to share my experience with you.

My first impression of the product? Neat and mess-free. Exuding an expensive and premium taste, the golden, honeycomb-shape drop does have a lot of novelty appeal. My "out of box" experience with the product was not 100% positive though. It wasn't totally easy to remove from the little plastic package as the base of the honey drop got stuck to the plastic I had to flick it out with my fingers. Perhaps, the weather here is so warm that the honey has turned a little sticky? I prepared a cup of warm English Chamomile tea, and added the honey drop. While stirring to dissolve it, it got stuck to the base of the cup and the spoon. But within a minute, all was dissolved.

What first got my attention was its claim of "the world's first 100% pure honey drop" since most honey candies contain additives such as sweeteners and starch-like substances for turning the honey into hard solid forms. I know manufacturers will never reveal the process or technology behind this, but a question did pop up and bother me, would processing and drying honey into solid form in any way affect the health properties of honey?

And the price? A box of 20 units cost about 10 US dollars. This means each unit of 5g (equivalent to 0.2 teaspoon of honey) costs about 0.50USD. This is quite a substantial amount for a cup of tea or coffee enjoyed at home. I believe many people would switch from using table sugar to honey for health reasons, but how many would switch from using liquid or cream honey to honey drop for the benefit of convenience (less messy)? Special honey varieties (e.g. UMF Manuka) do command high prices, but for regular honey, besides the up-scale market like the restaurants and hotels industry, I wonder how many regular home honey end-users would fork out so much for honey drops.

What's Honey Powder?

Is honey powder just as good as honey?

Like many of you, I was all curious to find out what on earth honey powder is when I first spotted it in the shop overseas (I'm not sure if it's available locally but I've never seen it here on the shelves before).

How does honey get into this form? Why isn't there even a hint of yellow or brown color but pure white if it's made from honey? Is there really honey in it? Could it be icing sugar creatively marketed with a different name? A torrent of questions shot through my mind as I tried to figure what this pure-white powder bearing the label of honey could be...

My Findings - Honey Powder Revealed:

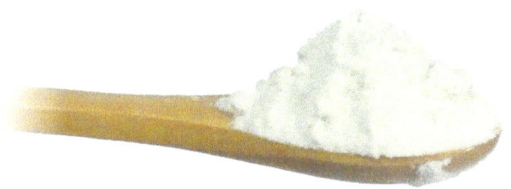

- Also known as dry or dehydrated honey.
- White and has a texture similar to corn flour.
- Sprayed dried into fine powder using high heat.
- Contains stabilizer that is made of wheat, starches or sugars such as maltodextrin and fructose.
- Commonly used as an ingredient in baking where the moisture content of recipes is limited. A one to one

ratio is applied when replacing table sugar with the powder.

- Also popularly used as a sprinkle on cereal, puddings, biscuits, cakes, and breads.
- Has the benefit of non-stickiness, mess-free, no crystallization issues, and easy clean up.

So how does the powder form of honey compare with liquid honey? You judge and make your own verdict.

What About Cactus Honey Powder?

I'm not sure how many of you have come across Cactus Honey Powder but for those who have, you probably assume it's a honey varietal from the flowers of cactus that's been processed into powder form for the convenience of use, just as how one brand has sold it - 'just scoop and mix it into your coffee and tea like you would use sugar or creamer'.

This honey powder is not sold in every country, but many suppliers of honey products in the World Wide Web seem to be carrying this product. Claimed to be all natural, this honey powder is marketed as all natural, healthy to eat, and an excellent sugar replacement suitable for the diabetic. And it's positioned as a brilliant ingredient for baking or drizzled on cereals, pancakes and waffles. However, I had all these questions in my mind: How can it be a product from the bees when even the lightest-colored honey cannot be colorless or white? And even if it is really honey, what's the process involved in making honey liquid into powder form? Are any health benefits compromised as a result processing?

Leading consumers to naturally think it's a variety of honey, the name "Cactus honey" is a misnomer. Actually, cactus honey powder doesn't come from the bees. It's made from the juice of a Mexico-native cactus plant called Agave. Like maple syrup and cane sugar; its juice after filtering is heated to remove excess water. The liquid form is probably a lot better known – Agave syrup or Agave sweetener, which started to appear on the shelves of health food in the early 2000s. This plant-based sweetener is more viscous than honey and is about 90% fructose, the natural sweetener found in most fruits.

Agave syrup is not as aggressive as table sugar in spiking our body blood sugar due to its lower glycemic index. However, in my opinion, it seems like one of those highly processed sweeteners which are often used in baking. Also, I find it hard to appreciate the way the product has associated itself with bee's honey.

Wild Guesses about Wild Honey

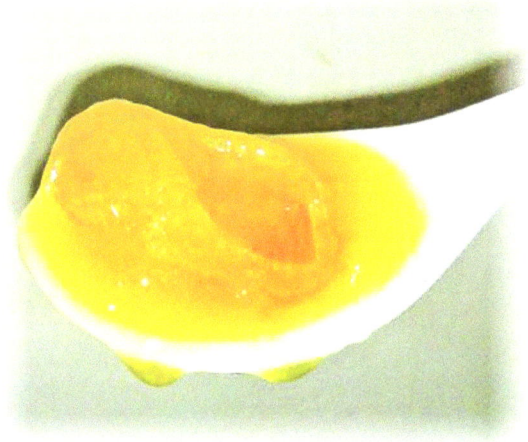

I'm not sure what you would consider as rare bee products, but some honey retailers are raving about honey from the wild, as in honey extracted from wild honeycombs produced by honeybees in the wild forest, as opposed to most regular honey farmed by beekeepers in man-made hives. This particular prominent honey chain has sprung up here in Singapore with its branches mushrooming over the island one after another quickly, selling a good variety of supposedly premium, high-end, exotic honey such as Mahogany honey, Kinghood honey, Anchovy Pear honey, etc., Claiming that their honey is unique and of greater value than others, the shop's aggressive marketing efforts include shop front direct selling, print advertising, and even TV commercials. Their claims can be summarized as follows:

"Unlike other honey, our honey is harvested from natural hives in the wild forests e.g those of Africa. They are gathered from drops of honey falling down directly from honeycombs and have bypassed all thermal treatments...Laboratory reports have established our products as wild honey, which has more superior health benefits than honey extracted form made-made hives. Wild honey has a very slight sour taste. And when mixed in water, the solution obtained is clear and not cloudy."

A further scan through of the information found on the packaging of some wild honey bee products helps to put together a summary of their retail claims:

Wild Honey versus Beekeeper's Honey:

1. The potency or health benefits of wild honey are seven times more than honey from cultivated bees. (Price tag of wild honey is several times bigger too!)
2. Wild honey is not as sweet and has a natural sour taste as well.
3. When mixed with water, wild honey is transparent and clear, whereas regular honey turns cloudy.
4. Wild honey doesn't freeze when refrigerated.
5. When mixed with wild honey, egg yolk would appear to become half-cooked. (This strikes a similarity with the common folk belief for testing pure honey.)

I'm not trying to put these wild honey sellers out of business, but my curiosity about where exactly these wild honeycombs are obtained from and how true the claims about wild honey are just wouldn't let me go. Does wild honey really taste sour? And does it produce a clear solution when mixed with water? Such rare honey must be difficult to collect!

Puzzling Wild Honey Questions

I got several jars of the honey to satisfy my curiosity. Each jar (600g) cost about 70 Sing dollars, equivalent to about 55 US dollars (a very steep price compared to regular honey!). Regardless of its appearance (both transparent and translucent varieties), the honey really turned out to be very clear when mixed with water. The honey was unusually clear candy-hard (as opposed to the expected thick but soft texture of creamed honey). Much to my frustration, it literally took me four to five minutes to dissolve it in warm water. And the taste? Generally pleasant, with a distinct sour after-taste. The shop has actually run a TV commercial before showing the results of the experiment, i.e. clear versus cloudy honey water. And this, I believe has impressed and wowed many.

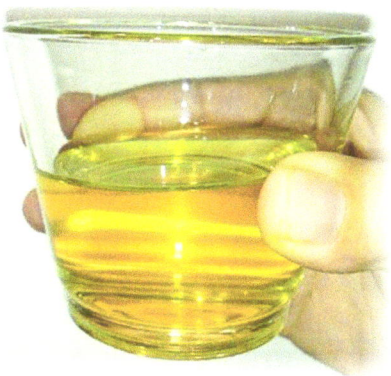

Some of their claims about wild honey have left me scratching my head. And I have also been warned by some beekeepers that the clarity of the honey solution could be a result of an ion-exchange process. After a few failed attempts in getting an answer to my queries from the seller, I figured that it would be a waste of time to continue pursuing any response.

Later I read in some online forum on the misconception that runny liquid honey means low grade honey. It explains that the popular belief, "pure honey is thick" (as opposed to runny) is an urban legend, and this has resulted in a lot of solid crystallized honey in the market. Other sources of information also point out that while different floral varietals of honey in different climates/environments have different viscosities, wild honey tends to have higher water content and less dehydrated as wild bees do not keep honey as their reserve food.

Don't Let Wild Claims Take You on a Ride

Check again, are you really eating real honey?

Many of you know that I love surveying honey on the shelves and in the World Wide Web. It opens my eyes to how much the so-called "real honey" is coveted" and "creatively" marketed all over the world. The following are what I have observed and my spontaneous thoughts on them. See what honey merchants are doing to cash in on consumers' lack of understanding on honey. Because there is no STANDARD for what honey is, honey labels and claims can get really wild!

1. "Creamy Honey"

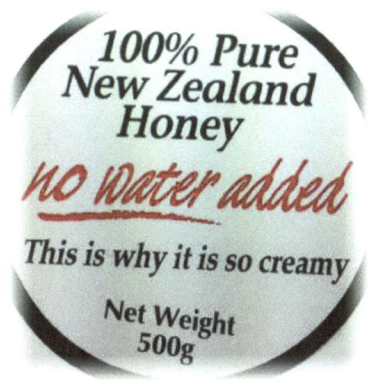

Being creamy doesn't equate to "no water added" or "100% pure". Liquid honey can be 100% pure too. And creamy honey can also be adulterated. Come on, honey merchants, educating consumers on honey is already hard enough; so don't add to the confusion please!

2. "Concentrated Honey"

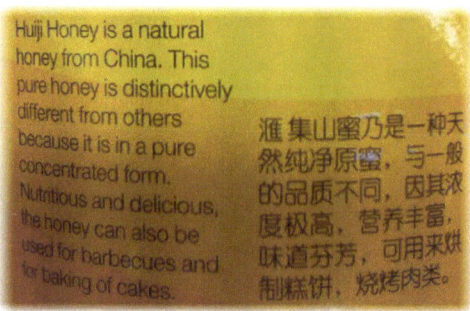

See if you can appreciate this whole string of descriptions - "natural honey", "pure honey", and honey "in pure concentrated form". The more the contents are described, the more suspicious if there's any real honey in it. Somehow, I just find that the term "concentrated form" sounds more appropriate for processed sugary syrups. What do you think?

3. "Honey Sauce"

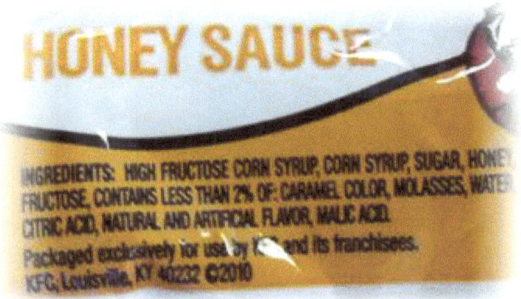

"Corn syrup sauce" would be a more honest name for this product than "honey sauce". Notice "honey" is not first but fourth on the list of the ingredients. It's disturbing to see how the number of ingredients has dramatically increased on just a teeny weenie packet of "honey". And I wonder if people have given up on reading labels because they have grown too long to be read?

4. "Honey Fructose"

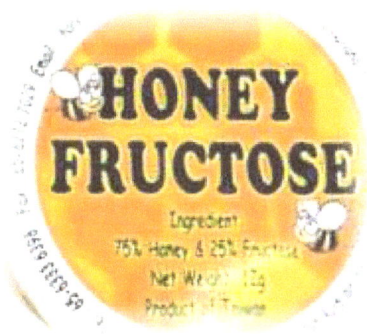

If people really know what "fructose" is, I don't think this supposedly healthy product can still stick and hang around. "Fructose" is literally translated into Chinese as "fruit sugar", which automatically sells well in countries populated by Chinese. Yet another high fructose corn syrup in dark disguise.

5. "Sugar Free Honey"

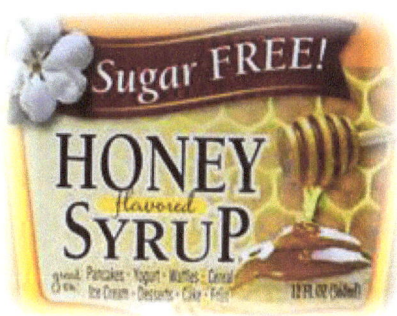

"Sugar free honey" sounds like one of the most ridiculous kinds of honey you can expect, but I am not surprised to see this, especially when the tide of "going sugar free" turns more and more aggressive. Its real contents? 0% honey and 100% Maltitol, which has been marketed as a healthy, natural sugar substitute for diabetics

6. "Blended Honey"

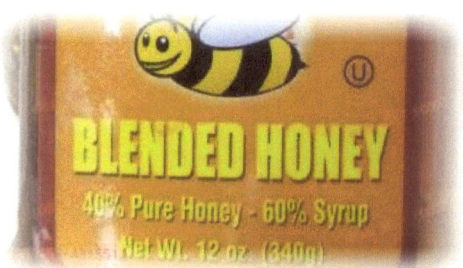

Looking at the proportion of ingredients - 40% pure honey, 60% syrup, you would agree that "Blended Corn Syrup" would be a more correct label than "Blended Honey". Well, of course no one is surprised, but I sometimes wonder how many people would enquire about the "syrup" they are eating.

7. "Honey Syrup"

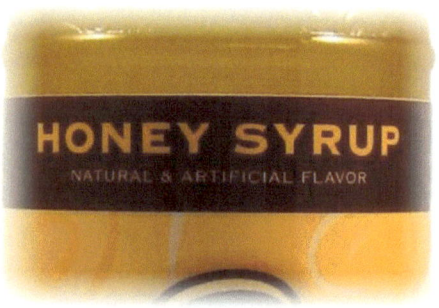

Oops, no ingredients listed on the bottle, just two claims "natural and artificial flavor" and "instantly dissolves

even in cold beverages" in its product description. Recognize how hard these sweeteners are trying to pit against real honey?

8. "Rock Sugar in Honey"

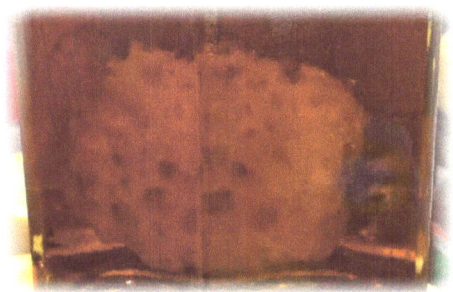

Just when you think that things can't go any worse with those honey jars in the stores, I found this one which made me shake my head for a while. For those who have never seen real honeycombs before, those pieces of those so called "Chinese rock sugar" would easily come across as honeycomb pieces. And the ingredient indication its jar label says "100% pure New Zealand honey". I just can't believe these jars of honey could escape the eyes of our food authorities.

Honey Purity Tests

~ Some of the Most Common Beliefs of Pure Honey

The following lists some of the most common beliefs of pure honey shared by sincere and enthused individuals. Are they true and reliable? By this time, you would have answers for some of them.

1. Pure honey is thick in viscosity.
2. Pure honey does not freeze.
3. Pure honey does not immediately dissolve in water.
4. Place a drop of honey on a piece of paper. Pure honey will not be absorbed by the paper.
5. Put a blob of honey onto a light colored round plate. Pour in some cold water to cover the honey. Swirl the plate several times. If the honey is pure, you would see a honeycomb image/pattern on the honey.

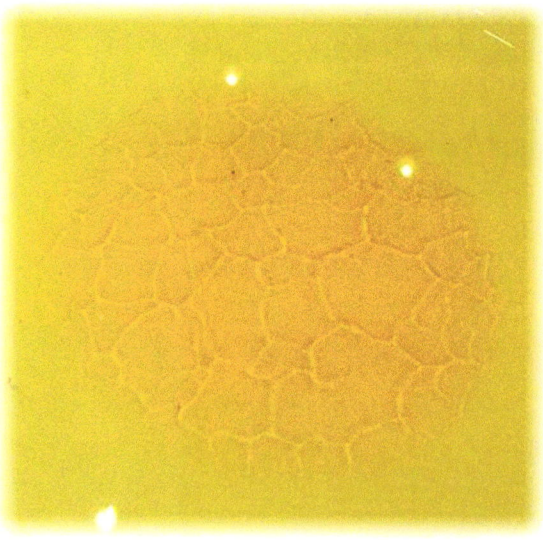

6. Cotton bud dipped with pure honey will burn when placed in contact with a match-stick flame.
7. Drop real honey on a leaf, pure honey sticks on the leaf like a gum.
8. Put some honey on a housefly. If the honey is pure, it will crawl out and fly away.
9. Pure honey is not clumpy.
10. Pure honey takes a long time to crystallize.
11. Dogs never eat pure honey.
12. Ants will not hover around pure honey.
13. Pure honey attracts big, wild black ants, whereas adulterated honey attracts tiny ants.
14. Pure honey does not foam.
15. Pure honey is marked by a pleasant aroma.
16. Check for pollen under a microscope.
17. Buy honey only direct from the bee farm or beekeepers.

Unfortunately none of the above test (1-16) are reliable. Tests 1-8 are related to viscosity of honey, which varies according to the different floral varietals. For instance, the phenomenon observed in Test 5 is not exclusive to honey, however fascinating and wonderful it may be. The same could happen to thick sauces such as soy sauce or tomato ketchup. For tests 11-13, many have found ants (including those tiny ones) and dogs devouring pure honey. Also, I could not think of a rationale why ants would prejudice against honey mixed with other sweeteners. Foaming as mentioned in test 14 can happen to honey depending on the extraction and bottling process. As for test 15, I've come across some artificially flavored honey types that are even more aromatic than some varietals of pure honey. The pollen test in test 16 basically tests for the presence of pollen in honey but does not guarantee that the honey is

100% pure, unadulterated. Raw, unfiltered honey will contain pollen, whereas filtered honey will contain less or no pollen at all, but this does not mean filtered honey is impure or fake. And finally, I totally agree with test 17, which is buying direct from the bee farms, but sadly in many parts of the world, you just don't have the privilege of accessing to any bee farms or beekeepers.

Get more stories on honey purity tests from people all over the world of different cultures in: www.benefits-of-honey.com/pure-honey.html. I know the conclusion that there is no simple test from home for honey purity paints a gloomy picture for the consumer, but honey can be unscrupulously adulterated in various ways such as the addition of water, starch, saw dust, chalk, corn syrup, and other processed or artificial sweeteners and flavoring, making testing complex and difficult to administer from home.

Does Real Honey Spoil?

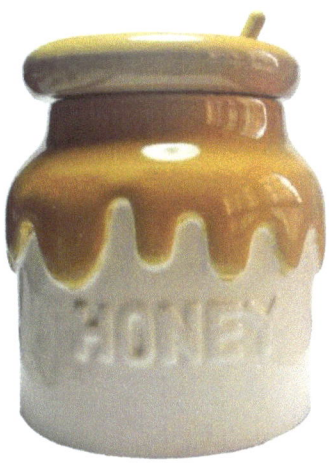

While one of the greatest facts on honey storage is that it doesn't spoil even with no preservatives and additives, liquid honey is susceptible to physical and chemical changes during storage; it tends to darken and lose some of its aroma and flavor. Over time, liquid honey also tends to naturally crystallize - a process where the honey appears to be thickened, become lumpy and grainy. Crystallization is easily reversible and does not affect the taste and quality of the honey at all, although it adversely changes its appearance. (So, please don't throw away sugary-looking honey, it hasn't gone bad!) For commercial reasons, a certain shelf life is often stated on the honey bottles in the shop.

For honey which possesses naturally high moisture content, yeast may reproduce over a long period of storage time and cause fermentation. While fermentation does not necessarily pose any health risk, some manufacturers do pasteurization whereby the honey is heated very quickly to kill any yeast cell and then rapidly cooled. A more common reason for applying heat to honey is to allow easy filtering of the microscopic particles and bee pollen, and delaying the granulation process of the honey (especially for certain floral varietals). This way, honey will last longer in its liquid state (and look desirable) on the shelves.

I often read about honey storage tips that honey has to be kept at room temperature and should not be stored in too cold nor too hot place. The problem here is it can be confusing because room temperature varies from country to country! For instance, where I live, room temperature sometimes could be as high as 35°C but I do not refrigerate any of my honey as cold temperatures would speed up the process of granulation. Also, the rate of crystallization varies for the different types of honey. Tupelo honey and Acacia honey, for instance, tend to stay liquid and is able to resist crystallization better than other types of honey, whereas Lavender honey rushes to crystallize. Honey that has been processed and heated will remain liquid for a few months.

Store honey in a cool dry place, ensuring that the container cap is on tight since honey tends to absorb moisture from the environment, which can lower its quality. Always use a dry spoon to scoop honey from the bottle to ensure that no moisture is introduced into the honey. Also store honey away from direct sunlight as it could affect its properties. This is the reason why some honey comes in dark containers. However, these dark containers do not allow consumers to judge the color, viscosity, clarity, and crystallization of the honey. Also, glass packaging is preferred by some people as glass is relatively neutral and doesn't react with honey and cause any chemical transfer. However, I don't see why plastic containers should be a concern if the honey is to be used regularly and not for a long storage period. It's easy to restore granulated honey to its natural state, for instance you could put grainy honey on hot toast, the granules will melt as you eat. You can also place a granulated jar over hot water (about 40-50°C), as soon as the granules are dissolved, remove the honey from the heat and let it cool as quickly as possible. Remember, avoid adding boiling hot water to honey!

Frequently Asked Questions About Honey

Below is a compilation of some of the most commonly questions received through our website, www.benefitsof-honey.com. These questions and their high frequencies of submission are enough to tell us how misinformed consumers are about honey and its properties.

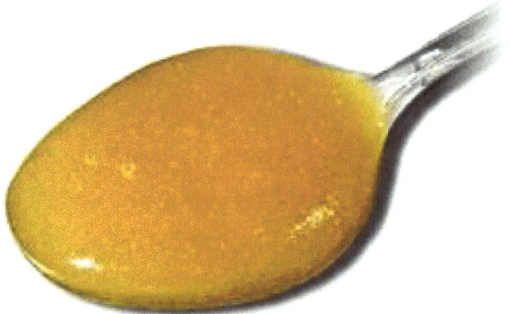

1. Most honey is labeled "pure honey", but what exactly does "pure honey" mean?

Pure natural honey is not diluted and contains no additives, preservatives, artificial or synthetic ingredients. It contains only one ingredient - honey.

2. What is raw honey and are all raw honey creamed honey?

Raw honey is totally unheated and unprocessed. It usually granulates within weeks. Few varietals in the raw form are liquid. Honey sellers and packers that face crystallization issues would cream their honey. But there are exceptions of course; some floral varietals, especially those in Asia, granulate very slowly, so raw honey can too be in clear liquid form. And most of the time, when you get unlabeled bottles of honey direct from small-scale beekeepers, it is in the raw liquid form.

(**Note:** While creaming helps to address crystallization issues, I believe it is also used as a marketing tactic to differentiate the honey from the rest of the honey in its most original liquid form.)

3. Is creamed or semi-solid honey more superior to clear liquid honey?

The creamy texture of honey does not imply any superiority in terms of quality or health benefits. Many marketing labels such as "nothing is added, that's why our honey is so creamy" have misled consumers to think the creamier the honey, the purer it is.

Creamed honey is formed by blending a specific ratio of finely granulated honey and liquid honey. The mixture is then placed in cool storage to promote rapid granulation and produce a small crystal structure that results in a smooth creamy texture. The precisely controlled crystallization process also lightens the color of honey (some creamed honey is white), but does not alter the taste or affect the nutritional value. The only difference in cream and clear liquid honey is the form and texture, nothing more and nothing less.

4. My honey has turned coarse, grainy and looks sugary and unappetizing. Is it a sign of adulteration with processed sugar or has it gone off?

Granulation or crystallization of honey is a natural process and does not affect the quality of honey. You can still eat it. Some floral varietals have a tendency to granulate more quickly than others and cold temperature also speeds up the rate of crystallization. To return grainy honey to its clear liquid state, simply place the jar over a warm water bath.

5. Why does my creamed honey darken and becomes runny?

Over time, warm climate or storage condition can cause cream honey to become darker in color, less viscous and runnier. The honey has returned closer to its original liquid state. Avoid placing honey near the windows and on shelves above the kitchen stove as high temperature can cause honey to lose its flavor. For creamed honey that is too solid hard, you can run the jar in a warm bath to make it runny again. As a general principle, warm to soften, cool to firm.

Many people erroneously associate dark honey with "aged honey" and an attribute of superiority gained over time. Actually, "aged honey", which is generally more intense in flavor, refers to honey resulting from aging and fermentation of the honey in the natural wild bee hive. This it is thus different from the honey that has been extracted and stored in containers for a long time.

6. I suppose all honey that is not labeled "raw honey" is pasteurized?

While honey that is cold filtered directly from the extracting barn is often differentiated by a "raw honey" label, honey that is not labeled raw may not necessarily be pasteurized (heated to about 60-70 degrees Celsius). Some honey suppliers only lightly warm their honey (about 40 degrees Celsius) for the purpose of easier straining and bottling and the nutrients and live enzymes are still kept in. But their honey may not be labeled as "raw".

Requirements related to pasteurized and raw honey are different for different countries. There are no legal regulations in the United States for labeling honey as "raw". It is possible for honey to be boiled and still label as "raw". Thus it is so important to get your honey from a trusted supplier. In some grocery stores, honey is required to be pasteurized to extend shelf life, but not everywhere has a pasteurization procedure for honey, in some places, pasteurization and heating of honey are not necessary; hence honey is expected to be raw. Whether there is any "raw" label on the bottle is irrelevant.

7. I was told that bacteria cannot reproduce in honey due to its composition, so why do some commercial brands pasteurize their honey?

Many people assume pasteurization kills bacteria in honey and hence in some places, it has become a commercial requirement for honey to be sold in the stores. While it is true that honey is pasteurized for safety reasons in some countries, it is not the same everywhere.

Pasteurization is also very much a marketing issue. Certain varietals of honey crystallize quickly and are seen as defects by consumers. Heating and filtering retards the crystallization process and keeps the honey presentable on the shelves. In some countries, I get puzzled looks when I ask the honey seller if their honey has been pasteurized. Obviously they find my question very strange because for what they know, there is absolutely no need to heat honey!

8. Why is the floral type (e.g. Buckwheat, Clover, Thyme, Macadamia, Manuka, Eucalyptus, Aster, Dandelion, etc) indicated on some honey bottles?

Honey that does not indicate its nectar source is also called floral blend, bush honey, or multifloral honey. Sometimes generic names are also given - wildflower honey, desert honey, mountain honey, Himalayan honey, winter honey, summer honey, Yemen honey, etc. The bees can forage a number of different flowers but the precise floral origin of the honey is not identified. Monofloral honey varietals are nectar collected by the bees that forage from one single or predominant source, resulting in a honey with its own unique flavor and aroma. Identifying and separating honey into distinct floral varietals can be a costly affair.

9. Is Manuka honey better than other floral varietals?

Hydrogen peroxide antibacterial property is common to most honey, but Manuka honey with an Active rating of 10+ and above contains an additional special antibacterial strength (Non Peroxide Activity) that helps to differentiate it as a medicinal honey from the rest of food-grade honey. (Note: Manuka honey with an NPA or UMF rating lower than 10+ is as good as regular/food grade honey.)

10. Brands can make a difference in price. But what other attributes could also influence the price of honey?

Apart from brands (which can have a significant impact on honey quality due to differences in nectar sources, beekeeping practices and beliefs and honey handling), other factors include whether honey is "certified raw", whether honey is "certified organic", whether it is a monofloral varietal, the abundance of the supply of that floral varietal, and whether it is a medicinal grade or food grade honey. Thus, there isn't a straightforward explanation to why for instance it is possible for two different sources or brands of Manuka honey Active 10+ to have a marked difference in price.

11. I have come across the term "local honey". What is it and where can I get it here?

Local honey comes from the bees that live in your neighborhood. There isn't a fixed definition to local honey in terms of mileage, but it usually means 5 mile and up to even 100 mile radius from where you live; the nearer it is, the better. As there is no honey production activity in Singapore, the so-called "local honey" does not exist here.

12. I suppose thick, high viscosity honey is better than runny honey?

Viscosity of honey varies depending on the nectar source. Honey is a reflection of the place (weather, season, soil, landscape) and flora the bees forage. Some floral varietals of honey are naturally more viscous than others. A runny honey may not be a sign of adulteration or production from sugar-fed bees. While honey may ferment more easily during storage and lose its freshness if its water content is too high, viscosity should not be taken as a deciding factor of honey purity or superiority in quality. Honey is hygroscopic, which means that it easily absorbs moisture from the air. Thus, in areas with a very high humidity, the amount of water content in the honey produced is usually relatively higher. One simple way of judging and comparing the amount of water (not purity) in honey involves taking two same-size, same-temperature, well-sealed jars of honey from different sources. Turn the two jars upside-down and watch the bubbles rise. Bubbles in the honey with more water content will rise faster.

13. Is the whole piece of honeycomb edible?

Yes, the whole honeycomb can be eaten and swallowed. The wax is made by the bees from the nectar. Many found the natural wax to be an excellent roughage, however most people still prefer to chew it like a gum and spit out the remaining hard wax.

"Honey is not just honey."
"Not all honey is created equal."

Erroneous Info-graphic That Went Viral

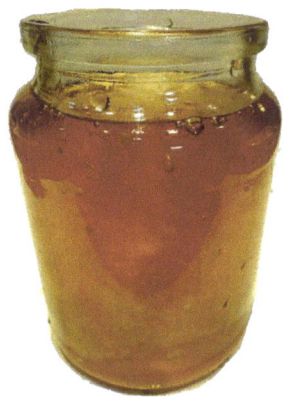

A huge info-graphic entitled "How to distinguish pure honey and fake honey" was spotted in a Facebook page that has registered close to 80,000 Likes. It caught my eye because it was riddled with inaccuracies and untrue statements and yet it had attracted almost 2000 Likes, hundred over Comments, and three thousand over Shares. It made the following statements about honey:

"Real honey causes a mild burning sensation in the throat… does not foam… does not separate into layers… has a nice aroma."

"Fake honey is sour in taste…is runny…is clumpy…has foam."

Perhaps it was created and shared out of good intention but the huge number of people finding the chart useful and expressing their gratitude for it was disturbing. No source or credit was given to the chart, but whoever made it had done a great disservice to consumers.

Firstly, I have certainly seen real honey from certain places separating into two layers - a liquid layer and a semi-solid layer. This is also often true of creamed honey when stored over time. Regarding the viscosity of honey, some floral varietals are much runnier than others, depending on the source of the nectar (flowers, weather, season, humidity, etc.).

In addition, not all varietals are aromatic. Each has a different flavor and aroma depending on the nectar source, some being more aromatic than others. A few even smell nasty! My first encounter with honey as a child wasn't great. I didn't know what kind of honey I was given but I didn't like what I tasted. And because of my first negative experience with honey, I was never interested in finding out more about honey until much later in life when I discovered that there were so many great tasting floral varietals!

Regarding honey being clumpy, most varietals crystallize over time and become sugary in appearance. Cold temperature further speeds up the rate of crystallization. Placing the bottle in a warm bath easily restores the honey to its original liquid state. I also have come across real honey that has foam. In fact several beekeepers I know confirmed that pure honey may foam. And to prevent the air bubbles from getting into the honey, they advise that the extractor be turned slowly and allow the honey to sit in hive temperature room before bottling. Honey should also be poured into the jar very slowly and poured as close to the jar as possible.

And as for why would anyone eat honey that burns the throat and associate the burning sensation with its authenticity, and which sensible honey merchant would make their fake honey sour, are all beyond me.

I've come across writings by apiculturists which instruct beekeepers on how to produce "award-winning" honey in honey competitions so as to boost their sales. And the criteria listed are often these – density/moisture content, absence of crystallization, cleanliness, absence of particle and foam, color and brightness, and aesthetic value. Going by these standards, the raw honey I bought direct from the farms (when I travel overseas) will never stand a single chance to be picked as a worthy honey by these apiculturists. This also explains why honey varietals which have higher glucose content and thus granulate more quickly than those that are low in glucose and high in fructose, are often creamed or heated to slow down crystallization. Also, being part of Asia, I have a lot of opportunities to be exposed to Asian honey (please don't immediately associate it to the contaminated China honey reported in the media). Based on those apiculturist' criteria, there would be so many awesome-tasting honey varietals in tropical Asia that will never deserve to be noticed due to its relatively higher moisture content and let alone qualify for an "award-winning honey" title. What a bummer!

Epilogue

If you have benefited from this book, get others to read it. So many others need to know the truths about honey claims and labels. Help pass the word around. While bee's honey may not be a big deal for most people but for what it is and can do every day for our body, it must be differentiated from adulterated honey, honey blends, other refined, highly processed sugars such as corn syrup and artificial sugars. I look to the day when consumers can stop guessing what they read on honey labels, buying a bottle of honey is easy and straight forward, and "pure honey" means pure honey and "raw honey" means raw honey on their bottles.

Cheers to a better tomorrow.

www.ingramcontent.com/pod-product-compliance
Lightning Source LLC
Chambersburg PA
CBHW050816290526
45792CB00001B/141